IMMUNITY SUPERHEROES

POWERFUL NATURAL SOLUTIONS & OPTIMAL VITAMIN DOSING TO STRENGTHEN YOUR IMMUNE SYSTEM DEFENSE

Allyson Haynes

Table of Contents

Huge Disclaimer

This information is intended as information and not a substitute for medical advice or care from a physician or a professional health care provider. It is not intended to replace medical advice. Medical care is essential for accurate diagnosis and appropriate treatment, including the application of information within this book. The author is not a medical professional, but rather is reporting on information researched.

The author and publisher provide the information in this book with the understanding that you act upon it with your own risk and also with full knowledge that health care professionals should be consulted for their specific advice before acting on any information provided in this book.

The author and publisher are not responsible for any goods and/or services offered and/or referred to in this book and expressly disclaim all liability in connection with the fulfillment of orders for any such goods and/or services and for any damages, loss or expense to person or property arising out of or relating to them.

You are responsible for your health and wellness.

Meet the Author

Hi, my name is Allyson Haynes. I am not a doctor or nurse, although I frequently get asked if I am one, as I relay health information to anyone who sits still long enough.

I will not bother to give you my life story since birth, explaining every bump, bruise, and cold I've ever experienced, which lead me to be motivated to learn all the information in this book. Here is a very quick summary and then we can get down to business.

Like most health and nutrition researchers, I started learning out of necessity. I was suffering from uncontrollable allergies and eczema, with no relief from doctors. After enough frustrating and fruitless visits, I stopped expecting doctors to give me any answers and started doing the work to find the answers myself. After finding relief, I decided to figure out how to improve other areas of my health.

A person who at the time would be considered a "health nut" suggested my allergies may be the result of too little calcium. Desperate, I stopped drinking coffee, and pop (I was drinking about 3 cups a day). I started taking calcium citrate and magnesium supplements 6 times a day. 2 weeks later my eczema left for the first time in over half a year. But it seemed to be on the edge of coming back all the time.

I went back to my health-nut friend to ask why the skin seemed so weak.

"How much Omega-3s are you taking?"

"What's Omega 3?"

That lead to my understanding of the importance of Omega-3 oils in my diet. I started adding flaxseed oil to my diet. Shortly after the painful eczema was gone for good.

That lead to an intense interest in improving my health using food, supplements and natural solutions that did not involve drugs. Since that time, over 20 years ago, I willingly invested at least 30 hours a week researching, reading and trying to understand as much as possible about health and nutrition, and natural solutions for health problems. I have read over 200 books and thousands of articles on health and nutrition, trying to piece all the information nuggets together. Even with decades of research, I still learn at least 5-10 new facts each day. Learning about how to improve your health cannot ever really be complete.

The difference in learning and implementing this research has been remarkable to our family's health. My 50-year old husband and I take zero medications and have no chronic health conditions.

We are extremely rare visitors to a doctor's office. We also look at least 10 years younger than our actual age.

We rarely get sick, and in the odd time that we do get sick, it rarely lasts long. Understanding not only what to take, but why and how much is needed has made a huge difference in our health.

Before you assume that anything in this book is absolute and that it should be written on tablets in stone, I want to be clear that I am not a doctor or any licensed medical professional. I have yet to sit through even one episode of Grey's Anatomy. If you are looking for someone with lots of letters behind their name and will talk to you with endless medical jargon, you found the wrong book.

So before anyone works hard to discredit my research, I want to make it abundantly clear. I have NO credentials. I am sharing what I have spent countless hours researching books and articles and cross-referencing to help you hopefully give you some powerful information in a simple to understand format. I am not selling any products or fancy funnel programs through this book.

Understanding all of this, if you want you to learn what I've found out, let's get started.

Introduction

In my experience, if you have a cold or the flu there are proactive ways you can help your immune system to overcome the illness.

It is a widespread misunderstanding that bacteria cause colds and flu. Colds are activated by viruses. This means that getting a prescription when you have a cold won't help. You need your immune system to rescue you.

Just because you are exposed to a virus does not guarantee that you will get sick. Look at some families where half or even all but one person gets sick. The other(s) were exposed to the virus, yet they did not fall to the illness.

If your immune system is working well, your body should be able to effectively defeat the virus with few if any symptoms. But, if your immune system is weak, it opens the door for viruses to set up shop.

If you want to get better when sick, it is your immune system that will determine if and when you beat the germ. Not drugs. Drugs may work to modify and help in situations, but ultimately your immune system must conquer the invader.

Your generally underrecognized immune system is quietly working behind the scenes to protect you from everything from parasites, bacteria, mutated cells, and all other foreign invaders, including viruses.

A Day in The Life of Your Immune System

This is what happens with a virus and any living system in a nutshell. The virus finds a way to enter the cell. Once inside, it takes over the cell, like an army overthrowing the government, and has the cell now working for it. The cell then goes into making copycats of the virus. After enough have been made, the cell will burst open and release the hundreds or thousands of viruses into your system. This happens over and over until it is defeated by your immune system.

When you get infected, your immune system has to:

1. locate the invader.
2. figure out how to kill the invader
3. transmit this information to your system so that all your immune system defense army has this information.
4. find all the other cloned invaders and then kill them.
5. Dispose of the dead invaders.

Once your immune system has determined how to kill the virus, it saves this information in its "hard drive", so that if or when this invader ever has the nerve to enter your system again, you can quickly have your immune system respond and kill it before it has a chance to do anything.

That is how amazing your immune system is. Without it, invaders would easily take over and you would not last long.

Keeping your immune system strong and able to handle its enormous workload is an important key to keeping you healthy. You do not have to just "hope for the best", and get rest when you are sick.

You can be an active participant in helping boost your immune system, especially when it is handling a virus or germ of any type.

This defense army needs all the help it can get to keep it in top shape and ready to protect you every second of your life. Show it some love. When you lose your health, you realize how important it is and how much you took it all for granted.

Understanding not only what to take, but why it needs to be taken and the optimal doses essential to strengthening your immune system is important as you take control of your health.

The solutions in this book to strengthen your immune system and overall health are simple, affordable and easy to implement. Now onto the supplements.

A Key Missing Vitamin You Can NOT Produce

Humans are one of only a few animals that do not produce their own vitamin C. We have to get it from our food or supplements. Without enough vitamin C, humans can die from a lack of vitamin c which in extreme cases results in scurvy. All other animals not only make the vitamin C that they need, but they can also automatically make MORE of it whenever they get sick.

For example, let's look at a little rat. Rats are reported to normally make 70 mg of vitamin C a day. But when the rat's body is stressed, the amount of vitamin C it produces is considerable- it will shoot up to 215 mg a day. There is a reason why the rat does not keep making only 70 mg a day when they are sick.

Whenever someone says they have a cold, it is not long before someone chimes, "take vitamin C". And then the person will say, I did and it didn't do anything. The next question, I ask the person is how much did they take today?

"Lots."
"How much is lots?"
"1000 milligrams"

There's the problem. They did not take enough vitamin C to give a noticeable boost to their immune system. They were trying to drain a bathtub using a teacup. If you want to use vitamin C effectively, you will need to take a lot more than 1000 mg. 1000 mg is 1 gram, which is less than a quarter of a teaspoon if you were to measure it out. 1000 mg *might* be enough if you were healthy. It is nowhere near enough if you were sick.

RDA stands for "Recommended Dietary Allowance". The rationale for vitamin C RDA of between 40-90 mg/day is the prevention of scurvy, but certainly not enough for optimal health. It also does not look at a person's needs when they are sick, older, or consider any other reason where one might need greater amounts.

I do not consider the absence of scurvy to show that I am healthy. A lack of one specific deadly disease symptoms is not the only criteria I use to determine my health status. Taking only the RDA means that you are probably still chronically deficient.

I am hearing that in China, the US and other countries they are using IV vitamin C treatment for some of their sickest patients. I would be surprised if they are providing only 1000 mg a day in treatment through an IV. Even conventional medicine is recognizing the importance of vitamin C for our immune system, and that minimal doses are not enough when you have an illness.

Dosage Frequency

Vitamin C has a short half-life. That means that it will drop out of the bloodstream and be cleared out of the kidneys within 3-4 hours. If you take 1 dose of vitamin C and only 1 dose, the blood levels will climb quickly within an hour, peak around the 2-hour mark and then drop back to the original pre-dose level within about 4 hours.

But, if you take another dose before the previous one can be cleared by the kidneys, your blood plasma levels will increase when the second dose is added to the blood level before the previous dose is fully excreted. You need to take the next dose within 3-4 hours of the last dose to maintain your vitamin C blood level.

It takes time for the vitamin C to diffuse into other cells. It takes time for the vitamin c to move out of the bloodstream and into the body.

The membranes of your white blood cells absorb vitamin C. If you want the white blood cells to be able to be strong, they need enough vitamin C. When you get sick, your white blood cell count also goes up, and so your need for vitamin C to build these additional cells also increases.

Let's look at it like this in simplistic terms: When you are not sick, you might need 1,000 soldiers (aka white blood cells) to handle any issues in your body. In regular times, those soldiers are on the lookout for anything out of place that needs to be removed – abnormal or cancer cells, viruses, bacteria, fungi, etc. To make some of these soldiers' armor (aka cell membranes) strong, they need vitamin C as a key ingredient.

Now let's say you just got sick. Your body determines that it does not need only 1,000 soldiers to fight the germ, it needs 9,000 soldiers. To make all 9,000 soldiers, all of them need the same need for materials as the original 1,000 soldiers. This means that more vitamin C is now needed in the supply bay to make the same quality and strength of soldiers or white blood cells to fight the bad guys invading your body. If you don't increase your vitamin C intake to meet the demand, you will still need to make 9,000 white blood cells to fight the germ. But there will be a lot less vitamin C in the membrane of each cell, which will make them weaker when trying to fight on your behalf.

In short, vitamin C strengthens your immune system by giving you the supplies needed to make strong immune cells.

Should a person take a huge dose at once? The short answer is no. There is a limit to how much the body can absorb at once. The higher the dose, the less is absorbed per dose. For example, studies have shown that if a person takes a 1 gram per dose, 75% (750 mg) is absorbed, which is fairly close in percentages. As you take more, a smaller percentage is absorbed.

At 1.5 grams, 50% (750 mg) is absorbed, at 6 grams 26% (1500 mg) is absorbed, and at 12 grams per dose, 12% (1,920 mg) is absorbed.

How Much Is Too Much?

Your body will let you know when you've reached to top threshold needed. That amount will vary based on the person and the strength of the germ you are fighting. Sometimes you can reach it within a few hours, other times you won't reach the threshold even after taking larger regular doses for days.

You will know you've reached it when your stomach starts getting upset and you have what is called "bowel intolerance" – when what is going out the other end is more liquid than solid.

When this happens, the good news is that you have finally reached the top end amount needed for this illness. But, remember that the kidneys will be flushing this out of your system within 3-4 hours. So, do not worry if the tummy is feeling a bit uncomfy; it should subside to normal in a couple of hours, and not require days to calm down. At this point, you can cut the amount of vitamin C in half, and keep going from there. You've got the level at the top end for the germ, but the need for higher levels of vitamin C has not been eliminated.

How Much Do I Take When I Get sick?

That will ultimately be up to you. This is what I do with any illness coming on, or I'm in the throws of it, I take between 2 grams to 4 grams at a time every 2-4 hours. I also take Ester C, which is a buffered vitamin C. I have found that this type of vitamin C is much easier on the stomach. If I take straight ascorbic acid, after a few 4-gram doses I can get stomach upset, but I don't experience that with the Ester C.

I keep up the extra vitamin C intake until the symptoms have all gone away completely, plus an extra day or two. Just because the largest symptoms have gone away does not mean that the immune system is not still being taxed by the germ.

The Sunshine Vitamin

There are vitamin D3 receptors in every cell of your body. That is how important vitamin D is to your overall health. It is one of the most important blood levels that you need to check and ensure are at optimum levels for your health.

Vitamin D is not a vitamin. It is a type of hormone that affects almost every cell in your body by regulating the expression of your genes. Vitamins are nutrients that your body needs. Hormones are chemical signals that are used to regulate or control cell behavior.

You need vitamin D3 to metabolize calcium and phosphorus.

THE BENEFITS OF VITAMIN D3

Vitamin D produces 200-300 antimicrobial peptides in your body. These peptides are produced in the presence of vitamin D to kill bacteria, viruses, and fungi. If you don't have enough of these being produced, you are more vulnerable to any bacteria, virus, and fungus, and in turn colds, the flu and infections. In short, you need these peptides to have your immune system working in top condition. Otherwise, your immune system soldiers are working with less than ideal equipment to properly protect you.

Research has shown there is a relationship between your vitamin D levels and how likely you are to get sick. The lower your vitamin D level, the higher the likelihood of getting sick with a cold, flu, or respiratory infection.

Some of the other benefits of vitamin D3 include:

- ✓ Helps in regulating blood sugar levels
- ✓ Helps in the development of the brain and nervous system
- ✓ Help in muscle strength
- ✓ Reduces cancer risk
- ✓ Helps in the absorption of nutrients
- ✓ Improves bone and teeth health (with K2)
- ✓ Responsible for the health of your immune system
- ✓ Helps to normalize blood pressure

Just glancing over that list quickly, it seems like, yadda, yadda, yadda, heard it all before. But, if you look at that list, vitamin D is an important part of so much of your overall health, especially your immune system. I do not want to do anything that would reduce the health of any of these systems, especially when working to prevent issues is simple, cheap and easy.

You make vitamin D3 from the UVB rays in sun exposure (not UVA rays). The sun works with your kidneys and liver to change the inactive vitamin D into an active form of vitamin D. However, if you are north of 35 degrees in latitude, this only happens in spring, summer and fall months. The angle of the sun is too low to stimulate vitamin D production in winter months. If you are in the United States or Canada or anywhere above 35 degrees in latitude, you should be supplementing with vitamin D in the winter months (November-March).

If you spend most of your days indoors in the summer months, you should be considering whether you are getting enough daily sun exposure to make the vitamin D you need. Sitting by a window does not count towards your vitamin D – the UVB rays do not penetrate through the glass, only UVA penetrates though. You need to be outside for your sun exposure to produce vitamin D.

The darker your skin tone, the less vitamin D you produce over the same amount of sun exposure. Also, as you get a deeper tan, the less vitamin D you produce. The as the melanin in your skin gets darker it inhibits the ability for your skin to make vitamin D. This also explains why African Americans have higher rates of vitamin D deficiency – they need more sun exposure to make the same amount of vitamin D.

Also, as you age, your ability to make vitamin D goes down because the concentration of vitamin D precursor decreases in your skin. The skin of an elderly person produces 25% less vitamin D compared to a young person over the same amount of sun exposure.

WINTER SYNDROME

The more you are overweight, the more vitamin D you need, as fat cells absorb vitamin D, which decreases the amount available for the rest of your body. A lack of vitamin D is also a trigger to your body to store as many calories as possible.

When the amount of vitamin D is reduced, it is a signal your body that summer is over and winter is coming (are you are in winter), which is the time that food is normally scarce. Your system goes into survival mode. Your metabolism slows and protects you by preserving every calorie you consume so that you can make it through the famine from winter. Trying to lose weight when this is happening is like trying to swim upstream in a very strong current.

Increasing your vitamin D consumption does the opposite – it signals to your body that summer is here with lots of food in abundance and that there is no need to store food in your hips and butt. So amazingly, vitamin D is a key component to influencing your metabolism. This deficiency as it relates to weight loss resistance has been dubbed by some as "winter syndrome".

Since only 20 minutes of full sun will produce 20,000 IU of vitamin D, taking only 1,000 IU or even 4,000 IU a day will not be enough to tell your body that you are in summer mode. Taking a smaller amount tells your body you are either in late fall or very early spring, which s when food still is not normally in abundance. So, you can see why taking only 1,000 IU will not be near enough to trigger a change in your metabolism.

Some common symptoms of vitamin D deficiency include increased appetite, slow metabolism, weight gain, poor quality sleep, snoring, restless leg syndrome, sleep apnea, muscle weakness, fatigue, weak immune system, allergies, asthma, cancer, flu, colds, multiple sclerosis, and depression.

WHAT ARE INTERNATIONAL UNITS (IU)

This is a term is a standard drug measurement based on biological activity. The International Units of vitamin A is not the same amount as the International Units of vitamin D. Instead of using milligrams, big pharma used the terminology

International Units. 20 mg of vitamin D is equal to 1 million IU (that is 1,000,000 IU). If you look at it as 20 mg, you would think of it as nothing. Changing it to a huge number of International Units encourages you to take less, not more of it, and creates a fear of toxicity.

Because vitamin D is not flushed out of your body as quickly as vitamin C and can accumulate in fat, it is possible to take too much and have toxicity, which sounds scary. However, vitamin D toxicity is very rare, and you would need to take super high amounts for a long time to get that level.

However, not enough vitamin D also creates serious issues. Just like too little vitamin C causes scurvy, too little vitamin D can create calcium deficiency and rickets. Like Goldilocks, you need to get into the right zone. The good news is that it appears there is a broad range in this zone before you need to worry. Since too many people either spend most if not all day indoors, live a northern climate where the sun does not produce vitamin D in the winter month and/or wear sunscreens full of chemicals that BLOCK your ability to make vitamin D, the odds are you are low in vitamin D levels.

FEAR OF TOXICITY

You can and should get a blood level reading on your vitamin D level so that you know where you are starting. They say that the best range varies from 50-70 mg/ml. But, from my research, you can safely go up to 100ng/ml or even up to 150 ng/ml without issues.

The concern with vitamin D toxicity is hypercalcemia, which is when there is too much calcium in the blood. Some of the symptoms of hypercalcemia include constipation, nausea, decreased appetite, peptic ulcers, kidney stones, side pain, frequent urination, confusion, dementia, memory loss, depression, pain in bones, fractures, curving of the spine, and loss of height.

The scientists who figured out what the toxic blood level for vitamin D found it was at over 300 ng/ml! Because of this concern of this happening, they led to a recommendation MUCH lower than the threshold. They decided through an arbitrary decision to keep the top end of safe levels at below 100 ng/m just to make sure no one went over. That is A LOT lower than an actual level of concern found in the research results.

While people are frightened of vitamin D toxicity and error on the side taking way too little, the research shows that vitamin D toxicity is *very* rare. Articles published since the late 60's show that vitamin D3 toxicity rarely occurs, even when taken at really high amounts. These articles were published because doctors were amazed that toxicity did not occur and contradicted what they had learned in medical school!

How Much Do I Take?

Do not take high doses of vitamin D without proper supplementation of vitamin K2! – more about this in a bit.

The general recommended dosage is not to exceed 4,000 IU a day of vitamin D, and in some sources, they recommend even less – sometimes I hear it is as low as 800 IU a day.

But here's the paradox: if you were to go outside at noon with your body reasonably exposed to the sun and no sunscreen for about 20 minutes, you would produce about 30,000 IU of vitamin D. The people in the Amazon who live outside make as much as 50,000-80,000 IU of vitamin D a day from the sun. So why would anyone recommend 4,000 IU and especially something as low as 800 IU as a top-end recommended dose?

Optimal Dosing

An excellent book for additional information on this is written by a Judson Somerville, MD, called *The Optimal Dose: Restore Your Health With the Power of Vitamin D3*. It is available on Amazon. I strongly recommend this book for much more detail. Dr. Sommerville recommends an optimal daily dosage of 30,000 IU a day.

What he overlooks in his book is the importance of K2 to optimal health and how it works with vitamin D in your system. It helps prevent toxicity, and prevent hypercalcemia by getting the calcium out of the arteries and into your bones and muscles. (more on this in the next chapter).

SUNSCREENS

Note that most sunscreens have chemicals to block UV radiation, such as octisalate, oxybenzone, avobenzone, homosalate, octinoxate, and octocrylene. These chemicals get into your system through your skin when applied. Sixty-five percent of non-mineral sunscreens on the U.S. market contain oxybenzone.

These chemicals are known to be hormone disruptors. Hormone disruptors have been shown to affect reproduction, such as changing the estrogen cycles in mice, lowering sperm counts in animal research, delaying puberty, and changing how your thyroid functions.

Sunscreens also use Retinyl Palmitate (vitamin A) because it is hyped to slow aging. However, the US FDA found that when retinyl palmitate is exposed to sunlight may speed up the development of skin lesions and tumors.

There are natural oils, butter, and products that can be used as sunscreens. I mix these with zinc oxide to make my sunscreen. We use our homemade sunscreen in intense sun exposure summer months without burning.

Zinc oxide – I use regular zinc oxide NOT nano-zinc oxide. There are concerns that nano zinc oxide can penetrate through the pores of your skin and enter your system. While zinc is good for you, zinc oxide in this form is not. Regular zinc oxide will sit on top of your skin and not enter the bloodstream. You can get it from a wholesale supplier of skincare raw materials, such as New Directions Aromatics. It's less than $20 for a kilogram of zinc oxide, which is enough to make MANY bottles of sunscreen. Since I only need 20 grams of a 4 oz bottle, one container of zinc oxide will give me enough 50 bottles of sunscreen.

The formula I use to figure out how much to use is 1% of the total weight of zinc oxide for every 1 SPF you want to have. This is not tested with any FDA facility, but it's what I use for my measuring stick. It has worked well for our family.

I then mix it into several different oils that naturally have an SPF, to give us a bonus SPF factor and help seal in moisture in the drying sun.

Below are some of the oils I use that have natural SPF. These include:

Coconut oil – SPF 4-5

Jojoba oil – SPF 6

Macadamia nut Oil – SPF 6

Shea Butter – SPF 6

Red Raspberry Oil – SPF – 25

Carrot Seed Oil – SPF 38

Wheat Germ Oil – SPF 20

It is not hard to find coconut oil. The other oils you can also get at a wholesale raw skincare store. Since you will not need the entire bottle to make a solution, store the remainder in the fridge to extend its life. Unless you want to start this as a business (which has a ton of regulations around it), get smaller bottles.

The Hero for Your Arteries and Bones

There is a vitamin that most people have not even heard of, yet is necessary to keep the calcium levels in your blood in check and to move the calcium into your bones and muscles. It is also a vital sidekick for vitamin D3. It is vitamin K2.

VITAMIN K2

If you are taking higher doses of D3, and even if you are not taking anything, you need vitamin K2. If you decide to start taking D3 I strongly recommend you supplement with vitamin K2. The rule of thumb ratio I follow is 100 mg of K2 for every 10,000 IU of vitamin D3.

SIGNS YOU MAY BE DEFICIENT IN VITAMIN K2:

- Cavities and other dental issues related to tooth decay
- Arterial calcification build-up
- High blood pressure
- Heart-related problems
- Weak bones
- Kidney and gallstones
- Symptoms of inflammatory bowel disease, like bloody stool, indigestion, and diarrhea

- Poor blood sugar balance issues and diabetes
- Higher chance of having morning sickness in pregnant women
- Spider veins and varicose veins

The K vitamin family are fat-soluble vitamins. There are 3 types of vitamin K - K1, K2, and K3. Each form acts differently in the body.

Vitamin K1, aka phylloquinone, is used by the liver for blood clotting. This is found in greens. Because K1 helps blood clotting. If you took it as a supplement and were on blood thinners it could counteract the effectiveness of the drug.

You can generally get what you need from your diet without supplements, assuming that you eat vegetables regularly, so it is normally not necessary to supplement.

Vitamin K3, aka or menadione, is a synthetic form of vitamin K often injected into infants at birth. There have been studies that show toxicity.

Vitamin K2, aka menaquinone, is vital to keep calcium in your bones and get any excess out of your blood. K2 is especially helpful in protecting your heart. It is more effective than vitamin K1 to prevent and reverse calcification build-ups in your arteries that can lead to heart-related problems. It is found in some fermented dairy products (like yogurt or raw cheese), fish and eggs. A larger list of food sources is provided later.

You can take K2 as a supplement. It is needed for your soft tissues, bones, and heart muscle. If you are taking D3 you should be taking K2. You can find this at most health food stores and on-line.

WHY IS K2 IMPORTANT TO TAKE WHEN TAKING D3?

Vitamin D3 increases the absorption of calcium and in turn the amount of calcium in your blood. You need K2 to take that same calcium out of your blood and into your soft tissues and bones and teeth. That means it helps to reduce the buildup of calcium in your arteries. By doing all of this, it helps prevent vitamin D toxicity as well.

D3 is essential for calcium absorption to get the calcium into your blood. K2 is essential to integrate the same calcium out of your blood and into your bones and muscles. This is important because if you have too much calcium in your blood it can build up and clog your arteries.

You need to allow the calcium to move to where it is needed in the body by having enough K2 and not just do laps in your circulatory system. K2 allows for the production of a protein called osteocalcin. This protein is made by vitamin D3, but it needs K2 to function. This protein deposits calcium and phosphorus into your bones and teeth, taking it out of your bloodstream.

There is a very large study, in the Netherlands, called the Rotterdam Study that supports the concept that K2 removes calcium out of the bloodstream. They followed more than 4,000 men. The results showed that those taking the highest amount of vitamin K2 also had a 53 percent lower chance of having aortic calcification and reduced their risk of coronary heart disease by 41 percent.

FOOD SOURCES OF VITAMIN K2

The 11 best vitamin K2 foods, and the amounts you need to eat daily to get 100 mg each day:

Natto: 0.33 ounce

Beef liver: 1.25 slices

Chicken (dark meat): 6 ounces

Goose liver pate: 2 tablespoons

Hard cheeses, (such as Gouda, Pecorino Romano, Gruyere.): 4 ounces

Jarlsberg cheese: 5.5 slices

Soft cheeses: 5.8 ounces

Blue cheese: 10 ounces

Ground beef: 12 ounces

Goose meat: 14 cups

Egg yolk (grass feed chickens only): 17 eggs

I am not a large fan of goose liver pate, and I have yet to eat 17 eggs in one day, let alone every day. Considering the amount you need to eat of these foods every day to meet the goal of 100 mg, you can see why supplementation is recommended.

There are 2 types of K2 sources. MK4 and MK7.

The MK4 source of vitamin K2 that can be made synthetically or is found in some animal product. It has a short shelf-life in your body and clears out of your system within a few hours. However, some will say that it clears out faster because it is more readily used by the body. But, because it clears out so much faster, you need to take it several times a day.

The MK7 source of vitamin K2 is made from Natto. It has a much longer half-life, so you don't need to take it as often each day.

K2 is a vital and generally unheard-of vitamin that is a key component to many aspects of our health.

Again, the rule I use is 100 mg for 10,000 units of vitamin D3. So if taking 20,000 units of D3, you would want to take 2- 100 mg   capsules.

The Immunity Boosting Mineral That Keeps Hair on Your Head

Zinc is required for your body to make over 300 enzymes in your system and often overlooked in its importance to your health.

Zinc is a key component of your immune system. It is needed to make a key protein, called fractalkine. This protein, which can be made in the presence of zinc helps the white blood cells stick to endothelial cells. Endothelial cells (ECs) are needed to maintain blood flow and prevent blood loss. If you want the white blood cells in your immune system to stick to the bad guys better, you need zinc.

OTHER BENEFITS BEYOND THE IMMUNE SYSTEM

But there are a whole host of other reasons to take zinc regularly, even when you are not fighting a cold or flu virus.

Zinc is the most common mineral in your nervous system. It is needed to make the neurotransmitter serotonin, which is what makes you feel calm and be able to go to sleep. You cannot take supplements for serotonin; you must make it in your body.

Now here is another great reason for taking zinc. The blood test for zinc deficiency is the presence of dihydrotestosterone (DHT), which is made when you are missing an enzyme that needs zinc to form. Why should you care about this? Because hair loss, such as male pattern baldness and female hair loss, has been associated with too much dihydrotestosterone in the body.

Dihydrotestosterone is a male hormone necessary in the womb. But when you have it floating in your body as an adult, it has no purpose.

So, it ends up attaching to hair follicles and blocks the hair from receiving the nutrients they need. When the hair follicles start getting weak from not enough nutrients, they eventually fall out. From this, one could see how proper amounts of zinc in your body could stop excessive hair loss and may even stop further balding!

DHT is also associated with acne, slower wound healing, increased risk of wide-angle glaucoma, joint stiffness, and an enlarged prostate and prostate cancer.

Zinc is also involved with your thyroid. It is needed to convert the inactive form of the thyroid hormone T4 to the active form (T3). Your thyroid is involved in so many metabolic functions, including your metabolism and energy levels.

A zinc deficiency also weakens the connective tissues throughout the body, including veins. This can create issues such as colon diverticulosis (pouches in the colon), cardiovascular disease, a weakening of the kidney structure, hemorrhoids, varicose veins and cervical incompetence in pregnancy. Other symptoms that come from the weakening of connective tissues are weak nails, poor skin, acne, spider veins on cheek and nose, Achilles tendon ruptures, bunions, fallen arches, groin and belly button hernias, and intervertebral discs.

Zinc deficiency in men creates a deficiency in testosterone. When there isn't enough zinc, it can not be used properly and the body converts the testosterone into other things, such as that dihydrotestosterone. This can create a testosterone deficiency.

When men have this testosterone deficiency, it can create depression, bone loss, muscle loss, and overgrowth of nose and ears cartilage. The zinc deficiency is a common cause of converting testosterone to estrogen, which results in man boobs, cataracts, and weight gain. This would explain why we see old men with large nose and ears, who are overweight with man boobs – it is all related to the lack of testosterone.

Zinc deficiency in women creates estrogen dominance. This creates a higher state of inflammation and creates symptoms such as sore breasts, an increased risk for breast, ovarian and uterine cancers and cataracts, and polycystic ovaries. The deficiency commonly results in the higher levels of estrogen converting to testosterone, which gives way to PMS, chin hairs and other hair growth. Plus, it then creates more DHT, creating the acne and hair loss in women.

The zinc deficiency breaks down progesterone and zinc is also needed to make progesterone, so a deficiency also interferes with our ability to make progesterone. Progesterone is a hormone that activates GABA receptors that balance PMS that comes from excessive estrogen that gets converted to testosterone and crosses into the brain. If you have bad PMS, it could be a sign of a zinc deficiency.

Zinc deficiency also raises your ICF-1 levels. Higher levels of ICF-1 are correlated with lower insulin sensitivity. Insulin insensitivity is where the body is less effective at getting the insulin out of your blood, which makes weight gain much easier and weight loss much harder. Both D3 deficiency and zinc deficiency will affect and increase your insulin **in**sensitivity,

Unlike vitamin D, we do not stock stockpile zinc in our cells in case of a rainy day. That means that even small zinc deficiencies can produce symptoms and a weakened immune system. That also means that there isn't an expect chronic overdose when you take the recommended doses. But if you take way too much, your body can help you out by vomiting.

Stress, alcohol, and drugs all use up the zinc and create a deficiency. Anesthesia from an operation and chemotherapy can also lower zinc levels.

If you are deficient, one dose will not correct all your issues overnight. It takes about 4 months of zinc supplementation to correct many deficiencies.

HOW MUCH TO TAKE

The daily maintenance dose is 20 mg. If you have a deficiency, 30-50 mg can be taken as long as it takes to reverse the deficiency.

FOOD SOURCES

Oysters, cashews, dark chocolate (cocoa is full of zinc), hazelnuts, almonds, beef liver, and meat.

To get the 20 mg of zinc a day, here is how much you need to consume from the highest zinc food products: (any of these, not all of them)

20 oysters

400 grams beef liver

400 grams sunflower seeds

500 grams cashews

500 grams of cocoa

600 grams beef tenderloin

600 grams peanuts

800 grams sweet corn

A Wrongly Vilified Mineral

That mineral is sodium. You might think it is strange to have sodium listed as an item to boost immunity, but hear me out.

The study that is being touted as the reason not to eat salt was published in 1975, and since then it has been cited in more than 560 articles. Here is what happened in the study. Some researchers found a tribe living in a tropical rain forest in northern Brazil and southern Venezuela who did not use salt in their diet and consumed less than 500 mg of sodium a day. This tribe also did not have hypertension, aka high blood pressure. From this, it was concluded that low sodium intake was related to lower high blood pressure.

What this study did not mention was that half of the tribe died from infections and parasites, and all of them had chronically high levels of C-reactive protein (CRP). CRP is a substance the liver makes in response to inflammation. The study also failed to mention that when salt was added to the diet of similar people in the region, it did NOT change the incidence of heart disease. This is in part because these people had a lot of daily sun exposure and high levels of vitamin D3, which is essential for normal blood pressure and cardiac health.

Sodium is necessary to help our body fight infection and parasites. Sodium is needed to act as an electrical current conductor for wound healing. If you are deficient in sodium it results in systemic inflammation, shown in high CRP levels.

Before you insist on having bland foods for fear of sodium, realize that your taste buds and body crave it for a reason.

However, highly processed sodium contains only that one mineral, and the goal is to have enough of all needed minerals in the salt. For over a decade I have used Real Salt by Redmond. It is unprocessed salt with over 60 minerals and mined from an ancient salt bed in Utah. It tastes awesome.

The Essential Thyroid Element

A long time ago, on the same planet as today, people lived by the sea. They grew their vegetables in the soil near the ocean and ate fish and plants from the ocean. All of these had high amounts of iodine. The iodine fed all our bodies and brains. This helped humans evolve to have smarter brains.

Then people moved away from the sea and more inland, as is found in North America. When this happened, they had less access to iodine-rich foods and fish. Along the Michigan area in the early 1900s, it was called the goiter belt because so many people were developing goiters as a result of a diet lacking in iodine. That was when the government of the day mandated the salt – an item that everyone would have in their pantry would have iodine added to it. This increase in iodine stopped people from getting goiters.

However, there was no minimum amount required to be added to the salt. Eventually, the salt companies realized that they could dramatically reduce the amount of iodine in salt and still call it iodized. Today many people are chronically deficient in iodine and have thyroid issues.

Your thyroid is a huge consumer of iodine. When they check your thyroid hormone levels, they check your T4 and T3 levels. The 4 and 3 is the number of iodine molecules attached to the hormone. Iodine is essential for proper thyroid functioning. Your thyroid makes hormones that regulate the activities of most cells in your body and have an important role in brain development.

One of the most common drugs prescribed in North America is Synthroid, used to address poorly functioning thyroids.

Iodine is also essential for your heart health, your skin and sexual organs. Researchers found that people with breast cancer had a low level of iodine in their breast tissue. The risk of breast cancer increased with low levels of iodine when there was also a deficiency in vitamin D3.

Iodine is needed for healthy skin. If you have perpetually dry skin, and skin cream does little to nothing to help, it can be a sign of deficiency.

Other symptoms of iodine deficiency include dry hair, loss of libido, brain fog and memory problems, difficulty losing weight (because the thyroid is related to your metabolism), feeling cold when you shouldn't be, perpetually cold hands and feet, and constipation.

Food Sources

Seaweed (1 sheet) 16 – 2,900 mcg

3 oz baked cod 99 mcg

1 oz cranberries 90 mcg

1 medium baked potato 60 mcg

I take a couple of drops of Nascent Iodine daily. It is an electrically charged iodine which is easier to absorb.

A Key Mineral to Handle Toxins

Whenever you take iodine, you need to take it with selenium. Selenium is needed for the proper absorption and utilization of iodine. Even if you do not take iodine, I still recommend selenium daily. Selenium is needed for your thyroid to convert your T4 (inactive form) to T3 (active form).

Selenium helps your immune system by helping your liver process and eliminate toxins. Your liver has a 2-stage approach to neutralizing toxins.

The first toxin elimination step creates a reaction where the toxin goes from toxin to a "super toxin". In the second step, the "super toxin" reacts with selenium to neutralize it and allow it to leave the body. If there is not enough selenium in your body it can create a backlog of toxins to process.

Selenium is so important to your health that well over a decade ago it was determined that people who consume 200 mg of selenium a day decrease their risk of colon cancer by 30%. Yet, despite this huge find, there little if anything mentioned in the media.

A symptom of selenium deficiency is having the skin on your feet peel.

You can find selenium in the vitamin section of any major store, at health food stores or online. You can also get 200 mg of selenium from 2 brazil nuts, which are a rich source of the mineral.

It is a fairly cheap supplement to purchase. Without fail, I take 200 mg daily.

The Immune System Vitamin Needed For Skin Collagen

Vitamin B6 works in your body to facilitate a large number of functions, being involved in more than 100 enzyme reactions.

Vitamin B6 is essential in the immune system. It is needed to produce antibodies in your immune system. Vitamin B6 helps produce white blood cells and T-cells for your immune system. B6 is also responsible for making hemoglobin and protein called interleukin-2 that works with white blood cells.

But if that wasn't enough of a reason to take a B-vitamin complex, there are a whole host of other benefits to vitamin B6. This vitamin is involved in hemoglobin production, which is a key protein to make red blood cells. Red blood cells carry oxygen throughout your body. A shortage of hemoglobin with leave you feeling tired easily.

Vitamin B6 is also needed to make the hormone melatonin, which makes you sleepy and helps you achieve a deep sleep so that your body can restore itself.

Vitamin B6 helps make your skin look younger and healthier. Collagen is a molecule that cannot get into the skin by a cream – it is too large to be absorbed. You need to make collagen internally for your skin. Vitamin B6 is an element needed to make collagen, which in turn will not only help your immune system but also help you look younger!

If you are very deficient in B6, symptoms can include a red, itchy rash that can appear on scalp, face, neck and upper chest. Another symptom is sore, red and swollen lips with cracked corners in your mouth. All these can be resolved by increasing your B6 consumption.

OTHER SIGNS OF DEFICIENCY

Pain in Extremities. A lack of B6 can create nerve damage, which can show up as burning or tingling pain in your arms, legs, and feet. It can also feel like you have pins and needles in those areas. This can also lead to balance problems and challenges even walking.

Ironically, these symptoms can also occur if you overdose on this vitamin, so keep that in mind if you are one of those people who go to extremes on everything.

Depression and Irritability. B6 deficiency can change your mood and irritability. B6 is needed to make serotonin and GABA, both of which help with calmness and feelings of wellbeing.

Muscle Spasms. As GABA is needed to keep you calm, if there is an extreme shortage of GABA, your brain can become overstimulated. This can be shown in muscle spasms or jerky motions, and in some cases, seizures.

Increased Homocysteine. If you are deficient in B6, folate, and B12, it can create high homocysteine levels. Homocysteine is a crystal-like structure, especially in high concentrations, which can damage blood vessels and nerves. High homocysteine levels have been linked with heart disease and stroke.

FOOD SOURCES

1 cup chickpeas 1.1 mg

3 ounces beef liver 0.9 mg

3 ounces tuna 0.9 mg

3 ounces salmon 0.9 mg

1 cup boiled potatoes 0.4 mg

3 ounces turkey 0.4 mg

Banana 0.4 mg

How Much I Take

Since I am not interested in committing to easting 90 cups of chickpeas a day or 400 bananas to get 100 mg, I take a supplement.

I take 100 mg of Vitamin B6 a day, through a B100-complex supplement, so that I get the full mix of all the B vitamins, each with a useful function in the body.

As an additional note, B12, which can show deficiency symptoms with B6, is often not included B-complex vitamins, and when it is, it at very low levels.

Because Vitamin B12 is difficult to absorb, higher amounts are needed. I take a 1,200 mg sublingual B12 supplement daily as well.

A Cold Sore's Kryptonite

Lysine is not directly tied to conquering a cold or flu, but it is very relevant to conquering cold sores and the herpes virus. There are many different strains of the herpes virus, which can cause cold sores, genital herpes, chickenpox, and shingles. All of them are not fun to experience.

Once you acquire this virus, even when you beat it, it just goes into dormancy, waiting for a time to present itself again. It can come back depending on your immune system at the time, over and over. You don't just get one cold sore flare-up in your lifetime.

But there is good news. Lysine weakens the herpes virus. I consider it herpes' kryptonite. Lysine is an amino acid building block protein that your body does not make on its own.

Cold sores are caused by the HSV-1 virus. This virus needs the amino acid arginine to multiply. Lysine helps prevent this replication from occurring by blocking arginine.

If anyone in my family starts feeling a cold sore coming on, we amp up the lysine to 2,000 mg until it is gone, which if caught early enough can be 2-3 days, max, with the tingling irritation gone the same day the lysine is given. For a maintenance dose, we find that 500 mg every other day will keep cold sores at bay.

I do not have any experience for herpes and chickenpox or the shingles and there has only been anecdotal stories of it helping. But if the HSV-2 and/or HSV-3 viruses function anything like HSV-1, I would expect it to make a difference.

If you are looking for food sources of lysine include red meat, eggs, watercress, carob, caraway seeds, cumin, coriander seed, spinach, amaranth, quinoa, and buckwheat.

A Cheap and Unusual Technique to Stop Many Viruses in Their Tracks

This is a VERY important and admittedly, unusual, section. But just because this is not commonly known does not mean it doesn't work. When I first heard of using this technique, I was super skeptical. But after I understood the rationale, I was willing to try it and it works like a charm.

Since that time, which was over 10 years ago, my family has done this hundreds of times with great results and no side effects. It is surprisingly effective against cold and flu germs. What you do is kill airborne viruses that are replicating in your body by putting hydrogen peroxide in your ears.

This is why. While your immune system is wonderful, it has one weakness. It can only protect you where blood and lymphatics fluid flows, which is *almost* everywhere. But, the blood does not circulate in your ear canal, so your immune system can't reach it. Viruses can often be airborne and can land in your ear canal.

From there, it is the perfect warm, protective spot for the virus to replicate or incubate to its heart's content. It can make thousands and thousands of clone viruses and get ready for the launch into your system. When it finally infects the rest of your body, it will go through your ear and down your throat, irritating your throat membranes on the way down, which explains why you often get a sore throat as you start to get sick. It is the virus going into your throat as it begins its attack.

When you pour hydrogen peroxide in the sink, it will bubble where there are germs and kill them. When you put it into your ear, if any germs or viruses are harboring, it will have the same effect. If there are germs there, it will start to bubble as it kills the virus if it is harboring there.

If you want to try it, here is what you do: Lie on your side and put about half a capful of 3% hydrogen peroxide (the kind you get in the grocery or drug) into your ear. (Have a tissue on hand in case any spills a bit and to drain at the end.) If the germ is replicating there, it will start to bubble. It won't hurt, it will just make light bubble popping sounds. It may tickle if there are a lot of bubbles coming up fast.

If it bubbles a lot and then stops suddenly, you may have run out of hydrogen peroxide before you ran out of the germ. If that is the case, tilt your head to the other side and drain the peroxide into a tissue and put in a second application.

Continue with the same side until the bubbling stops. Then do the same thing on the other side.

If you put it in one ear and there are no bubbles after a minute, the germ is not in that ear. You should still apply it to the other ear. I have experienced more than once a situation where one side had no bubbling action, and the other side went off like fireworks. The germ can be lodged in both ears or just one. Never assume.

Also, do not assume because there are no immediate bubbles that it is all good. Sometimes it takes up to a minute for the peroxide to reach the germ in the canal and you start hearing the bubbles pop.

Finally, if you have a sore throat and you use this method when the bubbling stops you should no longer have a sore throat. The throat was sore because of the launch of the virus. When you stop the virus army from getting to your throat (and in turn the rest of your system), the reason for the irritated throat is also gone.

If we use the hydrogen peroxide as soon as we get a sore throat, we will find that more often than not we are feeling recovered by the next day. Instead of making my body handle thousands and thousands of viruses, we caught it in the hundreds, and my immune system could take on the challenge much faster. You can do this at any time in your illness, but the sooner you do it when you develop symptoms, the faster your recovery from this method. The more viruses that have the chance to get into your body, the more stress on your immune system to fight it. This method stops the virus from entering the body but doesn't do anything for the viruses that already are battling your immune system.

If you are around someone who is sick or you are concerned that you may have been exposed and could be getting sick, you can use this method to check if you might be getting sick. My husband was helping a friend at his house who had a bad cold. We found out that almost everyone who came in contact with the friend was getting sick very quickly.

That night, as a precautionary measure, we put the hydrogen peroxide in his ears. Because he had no symptoms, we were surprised that bubbles immediately came up like crazy. We even had to do 2 applications in each ear. It took about 20-30 minutes on each side to stop bubbling. After we knocked out the germ, he never developed any symptoms and did not get sick.

We have done this hundreds of times, and if the germ is brewing there, it works like a charm. The virus goes not always build its cloning army there, but in our experience, it seems to happen about 9 times out of 10.

This is a very cheap treatment (a bottle should set you back about a dollar and provides hundreds of treatments). We have experienced this to be a very effective method to kill viruses if they are hiding out there and all without taxing our immune system.

The Reason Kids Love To Jump

Your circulatory system has a self-pumping structure to get the blood flowing, called your heart and cardiovascular system. Your heart pumps the blood out, into your arteries. It expands and contracts 100,000 a day, every day, with no break, moving 2,000 gallons a day of blood through your system.

Your arteries are elastic tubes that contract and relax to continue to carry the blood through your body. It carries the nutrients and oxygen into your cells.

The veins do not have a pumping mechanism but have valves to stop the blood from backflowing until it gets back to your heart. The blood in your veins is low in oxygen content and high in waste products that will be further removed from your body.

The lymphatic system, on the other hand, is a network that helps get toxins, waste and other unwanted material (including all dead cells, viruses, bacteria, etc.), out of your body. Its main goal is to move lymph, which is a fluid that has white blood cells and other key protective substances throughout your body.

This system is a network of vessels, that are similar to veins and connected to hundreds of lymph nodes throughout the body, where the lymph fluid is filtered. The largest lymphatic organ is the spleen, which filters the blood, controls the number of red blood cells, and helps fight infection. If invaders are detected, the spleen and lymph nodes make white blood cells to defend your system. If you do not have your spleen, the rest of the lymph system will work to create protection, but you are more vulnerable to infections.

Lymph flows in one direction, towards the neck. However, unlike the blood system, there is no pump to move the lymph flow upward. Your system depends on the movement and joint pumps. What this means is that for the lymphatic fluid to move, it needs movement to push open the valves and move the fluid through the system. So walking, running, jumping, etc., will get the body to move, and the impact of your body against the ground gets the lymphatic system valves to open and close. If you stop moving, the lymphatic fluid and in turn, wastes are stagnant in the body. This is one of the reasons people will feel better after going for a walk or run.

Another way to get the lymphatic system moving is with a rebounder. A rebounder (think mini-trampoline) is a very effective way to increase the movement of your lymphatic fluid and drain toxins. The up and down movement and increased gravitational load (g-force) opens the valves and clears the system without a lot of effort. You can do this with gentle bouncing if you are not comfortable with jumping and still get the system moving.

Even 5 minutes a day of bouncing can make a difference in getting that lymphatic system moving.

Other Immune Boosters

Do you feel you are getting sick too easily or frequently or are around sick people and want an added boost to your immune system? Here are some considerations for things that might help.

OLIVE LEAF

Olive leaf is known as a natural, non-toxic immune enhancer.

Olives and olive leaves contact a chemical called oleuropein. This chemical is believed to have antibacterial, antifungal and antiviral agents. It also doubles to increase the body's immune response. The level of oleuropein decreases as the olives mature and even more when they are preserved. However, the olive leaf does not experience this drop-in time and can help fight bacteria, viruses, and fungi.

ECHINACEA

This plant has been used as a herbal remedy for over 400 years. Before 1950, it was had a medicinal status. Many of its chemical components are powerful immune system stimulators. Then antibiotics became the popular kid on the block and the herb lost some of its shine.

A meta-analysis evaluation of 14 studies published in the journal *Lancet Infectious Diseases*, found that the herb reduced the chance of catching the common cold by 58 percent and it reduced the length of the common cold by 1.5 days.

The USDA Natural Resources Conservation Services reported that the level of echinacea dose influences immune systems. They found that 10 mg for every kg (2.2 lbs) of body weight, taken over 10 days is effective to stimulate your immune system. So if you are 150 lbs, it would be about 680 mg /day. If you are 200 lbs, it would be about 900 mg/day.

Research also shows that the effects of echinacea are more powerful once the cold symptoms start, which would make sense. Since this herb boosts your immune system, it would be most effective when an immune boost is needed.

This extract not only revs up your immune system, but it also contains components that help kill the germs. For example, 2 of the plant species types have echinacoside, which is a natural antibiotic that can kill a broad range of viruses, bacteria, and fungi. Three plant species types contain cichoric acid, chlorogenic acid and cynarin that ramp up your immune system by stimulating phagocytosis, which is where the immune system eats up the bad guys.

One study also showed that echinacea can boost t-cell production by up to 30 percent more than immune-boosting drugs.

Note that you should use caution if you are allergic to this family plant-type.

ELDERBERRIES

Elderberries are dark berries found in Europe and North America. They are known to be anti-viral and boost your immune system, improve reduced sinus issues, nerve pain, inflammation and more.

For centuries they have been used to help people with the flu. They contain strong anti-oxidants, such as quercetin, kaempferol, rutin, and phenolic acids to prevent cell damage.

They also contain flavonoids that have antioxidant properties that can help prevent cell damage. As it contains a high level of anthocyanidins, these natural chemical compounds can boost your immune system and provide anti-aging benefits.

A 2009 study found that flu patients significantly improved their symptoms when they took 4 doses of 175 mg a day (700 mg a day total).

Elderberries encourage your body to release cytokines, which are substances that fight invaders.

Even after the cell is infected, elderberry is effectively blocking the virus from replicating. Elderberries' antioxidants discourage viral replication by blocking a key viral protein that the flu virus uses to get into the cells.

MUSHROOMS

There are some immune-boosting mushrooms that you won't find in your local grocery store, but that have strong reputations to help improve the immune systems.

Some examples include reshi, maitake, and cordyceps. They are all believed to strengthen the immune system and help regulate your bod's defense responses.

Reshi mushroom (Ganoderma lucidumi), is considered anti-cancer and immune-boosting because of its mucopolysaccharides. These get into our cellular membranes and make the cells more resistant to viruses, bad bacteria and chemical components that stimulate tumors. These polysaccharides also activate the white blood cells to engulf and destroy viruses, bacteria and other threats to our systems.

Maitake mushrooms (Grifola frondosa) have high concentrations of beta 1,6-glucan. This 1,6 glucan is considered to be one of the most powerful known immune boosters and adaptogens.

For example, the U.S. National Cancer Institute (NCI) and the Japanese National Institute of Health laboratory studies showed that maitake extract and strengthens helper T-cells. Other research has shown that maitake stimulates immune cells, and increases their effectiveness.

As it relates to cancer, it protects healthy cells from becoming cancerous and helps stop or slow tumor growth.

Cordyceps Sinensis is one of the most valued fungi in Chinese medicine and is used to strengthen the body after a long-term illness. This fungi works to boost run-down immune systems, but can also calm out-of-control immune systems.

PAU D'ARCO

Pau d'arco (Tabebuia impetiginosa) comes from an evergreen tree in South America. The inner bark is used for immune support. Not all supplements use the inner bark, so if you want to use this, it should be checked on the label.

This tree bark provides a double whammy – it boosts your immune system it contains lapachol, which is a natural antiseptic that kills bacteria, fungi, parasites, and viruses.

TURMERIC AND CURCUMIN

A study published in *Immunological Investigations* proves that curcumin can increase white blood cell count by up to 50% in just 12 days. Research shows curcumin helps to regulate cytokine production, which can help conditions with chronic inflammation.

ASTRAGALUS

Astragalus is an immune stimulant and has been used to treat chronic viral infections, hepatitis, the common cold, and flu. It does this by increasing the immune response to the viral infection. It also increases the activity of the phagocytic cells (the ones that eat the bad guys), antibodies and improves how the natural killer cells function.

COLOSTRUM AND LACTOFERRIN

Colostrum is what babies feed on from the mother for their first 72 hours. The regular breast milk comes in after that. It gives the newborn additional immunity when they are most vulnerable.

Research has found that the colostrum from cows is almost identical to humans, with the immune factors more concentrated in bovine colostrum.

These immune factors help the body stay stronger against viruses, bacteria, and fungi. The colostrum also gives antibodies to several types of bad bacteria including E. coli, salmonella, rotavirus, Candida, streptococcus, staphylococcus, H. pylori, and cryptosporidia.

One ingredient in colostrum is a polypeptide that helps normalize your immune system, boosting it if it is weak and balancing it down if it is overactive.

Another ingredient found in colostrum is lactoferrin. You can find this protein in the body where is vulnerable to attack, such as the eyes, ears, nose, throat.

Research shows that lactoferrin decreases virus and yeast replication, and boosts the immune system. When you have enough good bacteria in your gut, they also help the body make lactoferrin.

You can find this in health food stores and typically come in dried compressed powder discs. You are looking for colostrum made from organic grass-fed cows and standardized to 40% immunoglobins.

Immunomodulators

Keeping your immune system is top order is not done by simply boosting it endlessly. If your immune system is over-active it can cause problems as well.

An immunomodulator drug is designed to make your immune system behave a specific way either through immunopotentiation (stimulating the system to respond better), immunosuppression (reducing the effectiveness of your immune system), or inducing immunological tolerance (stop it from attack one particular substance).

Immunomodulation does not aim to balance the immune system, but rather to try to control it to behave in a specific direction.

In natural healing circles, immunomodulators are considered to be substances to help your immune system regulate itself better, by naturally boosting a weak immune system or calming one that is overactive.

The goal with natural immunomodulators is to calm an overactive system and raise the immunity of someone with low immune function by increasing the body's production of messengers that control and correct the memory of the t-cells.

It is believed that they can train the immune system to function more up or down as needed.

Some examples of immunomodulators include colostrum, L-carnosine, ginseng, rhodiola, and astragalus.

Other Factors That Affect Your Immunity

Keeping your system healthy is more than just taking enough supplements. Optimal health also depends on your caring about your overall health. Every part of your system is connected, and impacts to any one area will have ripple or direct effects on other parts of your body.

Here are some additional considerations, for how to make your body and immune system work optimally.

Constipation. The colon is a key part of your immune system. If your colon is backed up with fecal matter, you are not doing yourself any favors.

You want the food you eat to be processed by your body and have the waste exit in no more than 24-36 hours. If you think that "being regular" means that you regularly poop every 3-5 days, you are creating a toxic environment in your body. Healthy people poop AT LEAST once a day, if not more frequently.

Taking too long for the fecal matter to exit the system can create self-toxicity, where the toxins in your waste go back into your body. This forces your body more work even harder to deal with any bacteria, viruses, or fungus, as it has to process and eliminate the same toxins over and over.

Ways to help to clear your colon regularly is to increase water consumption, increase fiber (the goal is 30 grams a day), and make sure you take enough magnesium.

I take one tablespoon of freshly ground flaxseed and a tablespoon of chia seeds daily to maintain a healthy colon. I put in in a greens drink, which gives me a veggie boost, but you can also put it in yogurt, ice cream, on top of peanut butter sandwiches, etc.

When I travel, the chia seeds and flax seeds go with us. This keeps our family very regular.

Good bacteria in your gut help you manufacture immune boosters. Your system is not an island that can function alone. There are (are at least should be) more bacteria in your body than the number of cells. That means you need good bacteria.

Bacteria help with the digestion of nutrients, needed to give your body the nourishment it needs to stay healthy. Taking a daily good probiotic can help your immune system. This is not an area to discount in importance. Good health means working to improve all the workers in your system, including the little guys.

Diet is also key. Junk food has that label for a reason. When you are hungry, your body is craving nourishment, not empty calories. When you are deficient in nutrients, your entire body sees the effects, including your immune system.

You simply cannot make the same quality cells from chips and pop as you would from giving your body fruits and vegetables to work with.

My Immune Support Supplement List

This is the list of supplements I take every day to stay healthy for my immune system. Use this list at your discretion.

- Vitamin D3 30,000 IU
- Vitamin K2 300 mg
- Zinc 30 mg
- Vitamin C (ester) 2,000 mg morning, 2,000 mg night. Increase to 4,000 mg every 3 hours when sick until bowel intolerance is reached.
- Iodine (nascent) 5 drops
- Selenium 200 mg
- B100-complex
- B12 1,200 mg
- Vitamin E, mixed natural sources only (not synthetic), 400 IU
- Lysine 500 mg every other day. 2,000 mg/day with any onset of cold sore until clears. (I find that with the daily maintenance, the cold sores would stay at bay. It is only when someone gets lazy and stops taking the maintenance amount that we get a cold sore to deal with.)
- 1 tablespoon chia seeds
- 1 tablespoon flax seeds
- 1 probiotic supplement

I rarely get sick, which I believe is a result of actions and commitment to stay healthy. On the rare occasion that I do feel sick, and was not able to catch it quickly with hydrogen peroxide, I will also take one or more of the other immune boosters listed in this book.

This was a lot of information to process, and I wish you the best moving forward and taking control to strengthen your immune system.

If you are looking for more details on anything in this book, please check the reference section.

Thank you for reading this book and caring about your health. You have the control to decide how you treat your body and your immune system. Taking proactive steps to keep it in top order is easier than trying to manage a weak immune system in an illness. You can do this.

I wish you well.

Resources & More Information

Vitamin C: The Real Story. The Remarkable and Controversial Healing Factor.2008. Steve Hickey and Andrew Saul. Basic Health Publications Inc.

https://www.ncbi.nlm.nih.gov/pubmed/1584207

https://www.ncbi.nlm.nih.gov/pubmed/25023192

https://www.ncbi.nlm.nih.gov/pmc/articles/PMC5654973/

https://www.ncbi.nlm.nih.gov/pubmed/20536778

https://www.ncbi.nlm.nih.gov/pubmed/8155489

https://www.ncbi.nlm.nih.gov/pubmed/9644092

https://www.ncbi.nlm.nih.gov/pubmed/28863031

Sircus, Mark. Transdermal Magnesium Therapy: a New Modality for the Maintenance of Health. IUniverse, 2011.

https://www.ncbi.nlm.nih.gov/pmc/articles/PMC5579607/

articles.mercola.com/sites/articles/archive/2011/06/06/do-you-know-which-sunscreen-products-to-avoid.aspx

The Miraculous Results of Extremely High Doses of vitamin D3. 2014. Jeff T. Bowles. Jeff T Bowles Publishing LLC.

articles.mercola.com/sites/articles/archive/2010/11/22/the-common-cold-simple-strategies-for-prevention-and-treatment.aspx

draxe.com/nutrition/vitamin-k2

arganoildirect.com/the-truth-about-red-rasberry-seed-oil-spf-values-for-oils

thenakedchemist.com/natural-sunscreen-ingredients/

wholehealthsource.blogspot.com/2008/06/vitamin-k2-menatetrenone-mk-4.html

Vitamin D3, Zinc, and Magnesium: How to Prevent Many of the Current Health Epidemics (Dr. Jeffers Book 2). Asin B07N43H4S2

www.dihydrotestosterone.org

Olive Leaf Extract: The Mediterranean Healing Herb (Live Healthy Now). 2015. Lori Barrett. Healthy Living Productions.

www.turmeric.com/turmeric-health/650-inflammation-your-immune-system/turmeric-effects-on-regulating-immune-system-response/2538-cytokines

The Optimal Dose: Restore Your Health With the Power of vitamin D3. 2018. Judson Somerville MD. Big Bend Press

www.webmd.com/heart-disease/guide/how-heart-works

www.livescience.com/26983-lymphatic-system.html

www.healthline.com/nutrition/lysine-benefits

healthfully.com/274365-l-lysine-and-shingles.html

https://health.clevelandclinic.org/3-vitamins-best-boosting-immunity/

https://www.vitamindeals.info/articles/vitamin-b.html

https://www.healthline.com/nutrition/vitamin-b6-deficiency-symptoms

One Last Thing...

If you enjoyed this book or found it useful I'd be very grateful if you'd post a short review on Amazon.

Your support does make a difference and I read all the reviews personally so I can get your feedback and make this book even better.

Thank you again for reading this book. I hope you learned some new information that will improve your life going forward.

You are awesome!

Printed in Great Britain
by Amazon

16453338R00047